Printed in the United States of America

ISBN 978-1537572451

"In order to truly fight sexual violence you must attack the desire to become sexually violent, not the sexually violent behavior."

– Shawn Francis-Coleman, MS PC

Acknowledgements

I am extremely grateful to my parents for raising me with structure, love, support, and protection. I am particularly grateful to my father for the values and morals that he instilled in me; some of which I strayed away from during my younger days, but made my way back to. I do not ever plan to separate from them again pops. I truly appreciate Dr. Ian Edwards for the countless conversations and reflections that we share about life. If it were not for his sovereign style of discussion, I may not have recognized some of the talents and skills that I possess today. He is a true human being and one of the salient inspirations in my life that incited my passion to contribute to the fight against sexual violence. I would like to acknowledge all of the victims of sexual violence because far too often you have not been validated. I respect you. You are strong and powerful even if you may not be aware of it. I respect you and I pray that you realize that your life matters. Thank you to the organizations and people around the world who have and continue to hire my company to facilitate discussion seminars. I am indebted to you for choosing to partner with PerspectVe LLC and provide us a platform to bring great value to your establishment that you embed into your culture. We are passionate about this fight and standing beside you in the battlefield in the war against sexual violence is a true honor to me. To the readers, I thank you for allowing me to share these moments of your life with you. Finally, I thank the Higher Power for the blessings of my life purposes!

Contents

Introduction..pg. 09

Chapter 1 – Social Responsibility Vs. The Culture of

Concealment...pg. 13

Chapter 2 – Manhood...pg. 27

       BEING YOUNG...pg. 28

       WHO TOLD YOU THAT? ....pg. 31

       BEING IN-LUST vs. BEING IN-LOVE...........pg. 33

       SLUTS & BITCHES.......................................pg. 35

Chapter 3 – Can you tell I'm a predator/perpetrator? ....pg. 39

Chapter 4 – SIGHT AND SEX – *Talking to the sexual*

       predator...pg. 43

Bonus Chapter I – REDEFINING MANHOOD; *Addressing*

       sexual violence and rape culture in a way no one else

       will. ....pg. 51

Bonus Chapter II – Is It Humane to RAPE Someone?........pg. 55

INTRODUCTION

The more conscious I have become over the years the more I have been disgusted with the state of masculinity and the maladaptive behaviors it has pervaded the universe with and the negative impact it has had in the world. I feel the same way regarding certain aspects of femininity. In expressing my repugnance with parts of masculinity and femininity, I am expressing my dissatisfaction with humanity. We have not adequately, appropriately, and/or honestly offered ourselves or posterity a foundation for healthy maleness and femaleness because it has not been offered to us. Author Paul Kirby talks about how being male is not necessarily a biological construct as much as it is a social/political concept. I love when author and social worker Virginia Satir provides the idea that we cannot define what it means to be a man or a woman because we have not defined what it means to be a person.

I have a strong distaste for sexual violence and I decided a long time ago that I was going to contribute in the fight to kill it. One of the reasons that led me to taking action was not simply my abhorrence of sexual violence itself. I have sat on panel after panel discussing sexual violence, I have attended a multitude of sexual violence awareness and Title IX trainings and I am completely appalled with how some people are fighting the fight against sexual violence. A true problem in fighting sexual violence is within the vision and perception of many advocates against sexual violence. If you take a close look at cultures that engage in sexual violence, you may notice that a key element in the continuation of these unhealthy cultural practices are people and things that one cannot see and cannot report. The orchestrators of these evil cultures remain hidden (sometimes in the public eye) and the desires to sexually assault and violate people are difficult to detect in people. If one were able to identify these two elements then the war against sexual violence would be much easier to win. The problem is that many of the proponents to end sexual violence are fighting a battle against someone they cannot see and not paying enough attention to the red flags in predatory behaviors.

The majority of panels and trainings that I have attended are centered on reporting as many facts as possible and telling audiences how bad sexual violence is. I have no intention to saturate your mind with statistics that you may already be aware of and can find in other texts. I do not feel the need to convince you that sexual violence is bad. If you do not already realize that, maybe you need to go to some of the traditional panels and trainings out there that are offered. My goal in writing this book is to solely focus on how to kill sexual violence with effective solutions that have been ignored by the masses. I was at one particular training about human trafficking and the lady spoke in depth about all of the money that was being spent by the government to save victims of human sex trafficking. When I asked her how much money was being spent to address the root issue, which I believe is the desire to violate and victimize people, she said *none*. That is when I realized the fight against sexual violence was not being fought with a strategy to win. Though I am not in agreement with many of the ways that sexual violence is fought in America, I do think that bystander intervention programs are moving in the right direction to improve the culture but they still need to do better as well. "Currently, there are few interventions whose effectiveness has been proven through well designed studies.

More resources are needed to strengthen the prevention of intimate partner and sexual violence, including primary prevention, i.e. <u>stopping it from happening in the first place</u>," (WHO, 2016). This book will provide a strategy to win. Furthermore, I have seen far too often that sexual violence awareness programs are ineffective because they are created and driven by compliance. This book has been written not only to prevent sexual violence, it was specifically created to explore effective solutions to **killing it**.

<u>Social Responsibility Vs. The Culture of Concealment</u>

The first time I heard the term *social responsibility* used was during a staff meeting for a non-profit agency I worked for around 2013-2014. The agency was beginning to incorporate *another new model* for us mental health clinicians to get along better with one another in order to *make the world a better place.* Imagine that...the same people who spend large portions of their lives going to school to learn how to help people are the same people who need to be taught and reminded of how to get along with one another. But that's another book. The model being implemented was The Sanctuary Model® which was created by Dr. Sandra L. Bloom. It "...represents a theory-based, trauma-informed, trauma-responsive, evidence-supported, whole culture approach that has a clear and structured methodology for creating or changing an organizational culture," (The Sanctuary Model, 1985-2016). The mission of the Sanctuary Model encompasses teaching people and organizations how to form nonviolent cultures that are saturated with peace. As I learned more about the Sanctuary Model I was fascinated with it. Not because it was anything new to me but because it displayed a structured ideology of how I lived my life for the most part. The Sanctuary Model encourages cultures to make seven commitments for optimal health. Those commitments are *nonviolence, emotional intelligence, social learning, democracy, open communication, growth and change,* and *social responsibility.* The idea of social responsibility is simple. For example, if a group of people are walking down the street and they witness someone trying to break into a car, the Sanctuary Model would encourage the group members to take some form of moral action to stop the event. If the group took that action they would be displaying *social responsibility.* In the 1980's there was a serial killer terrorizing Southern California and when they found out who he was they released a picture of him to the media. The next day a group of people spotted him trying to break into a car to flee the area. The group immediately attacked him and nearly beat him to death. Though this is an extreme example, it is another example of social responsibility.

If you have not ever heard of the phrase culture of concealment, it can be condensed to the idea of the active practice in which cultures hide certain things. For example, some of the more notorious instances where the media has exposed cultures of concealment involve unlawful policing, sexual misconduct within sports teams and catholic firmaments, racism in the workplace, etc. There is a deliberate effort to protect and continue unhealthy practices to the benefit of manipulative regimes that turn people into victims. For example, "analysis of masculine collectives, such as the military or street gangs, suggests that there are indeed ways in which such groups promote and produce rape," (Kirby, 2012). Furthermore, "...Feminist have consistently stressed the connection of rape and sexual violence to other forms of gendered power on a continuum that encompasses many more areas of social existence," (Kirby, 2012). Another prominent example of efforts to continue these cultures of concealment are the STOP SNITCHING campaigns that have flared up at different times in the black urban community. It can be a challenge at times to expose, penetrate, and eliminate these cultures of concealment because of some of the ways they are orchestrated. Due to the fact that these types of cultures are based on *perceived power* and manipulation, there is a need for the regime to move in stealth, off the radar but heavily influential of the switchboard. Though these cultures exist in the physical with physical ramifications that hurt people, *the switchboard* itself is controlled verbally and mentally, off the radar, making it difficult for people against these cultures to know who they are fighting against. It is like being in a war zone filled with hidden snipers; even though you may have an idea of who they are (snipers), and what they are capable of (killing), you do not have as strong of an idea as to where they are.

There are situations in which cultures of concealment do show up on paper and within documentation. They are in clear view of everyone to see but they are concealed in the style of <u>language</u> and/or <u>visuals</u> being used. For example, when employers who only hire people with certain qualifications such as a specific degree and grade point average (GPA), they are actively engaging in and contributing to a culture of concealment; whether it is being done consciously or unconsciously. You may say *'Oh, that's bullshit. It's ok for employers to do that because they only want people who are educated.'* Exactly. I like the idea of what education could be but some parts of the educational system are gold members within the culture of concealment. It is called socialization. Before a baby is brought into the world, depending on where the baby lives, how much income the family of the baby has, the race of the child, etc., there is already a plan in place that will try to influence and determine the lifestyle of the child. The point here is that when cultures of concealment decide that they are going to live among the people while still remaining hidden, a new strategy must be incorporated and language is a great tool to do that. Words like *education, medicine,* and *employment* have been some of the great words and areas of life that have been promoted to help people while concealing the things that will hurt people to the gain of someone you cannot see (the sniper). The same thing happens in movies as well. One of the greatest places to hide truths, images, and messages, is in a movie because people will say *It's Hollywood. It's just a movie.*

I am not totally against cultures of concealment. Sometimes you must conceal things for the *benefit of people other than yourself.* For example, two past clients of mine in my private practice were very rich and they did not inform their children of their wealth until the children were much older. The parents had a belief (whether it was accurate or not) that their kids may become spoiled and unappreciative monsters if they knew of all of the money their parents had. Instead of making their children aware of the family wealth, they withheld the information, lived visibly modestly, and splurged behind the scenes. The information was concealed to the benefit of someone else, not themselves. That is the difference. The issue I have is with cultures of concealment like the ones I have been previously discussing; religious entities, educational institutions, sports teams, etc. I do not have a problem with the actual entities themselves, I have an issue with the things they conceal and/or allow to be concealed that perpetually hurt other people. I have a huge respect for Greek organizations on college campuses because I genuinely love the solidarity and brotherhood that they promote and actively live out for their entire lifetime. I love that. I must also say that just because I have an issue with how some entities, organizations, institutions, and beings in general who engage in immoral practices, it does not mean that I am against them ALL. I am not. I do not judge my interactions with person B based on my interactions with person A. Person A may just be a shitty individual and that has nothing to do with person B. So when I talk about educational systems, sports, etc., I am not speaking of any particular entity as a whole. When it comes to Greek Life on college campuses, there have been some isolated fraternities and sororities that have engaged in sexual violence and have promoted and protected the act of sexual violence within their establishment. This leads me to ask, *what is social responsibility within a culture of concealment*? One may argue that it could be the social responsibility to continue the regime as it is. Even though there is a small percentage of males committing sexually violent acts on college campuses, they are doing a large amount of the damage. The size of a negative culture does matter but all of them are still unhealthy. Even the smallest of subcultures within a culture can be hard to change. Scott McClellan writes:

> *"[It can be difficult] to change a negative culture that*
> *has grown up in an institution over time. No matter*

how obvious it may be that change is needed, and no matter how hard people of goodwill fight to create that change, social inertia and the selfish motivations of a few individuals who benefit from the existing regime make systemic reform very challenging," (McClellan, 2008).

That is true but change and improvement are very possible. Especially improvement. I do not like the idea of change as much as I do improvement. Change can be subjective and Pollyanna but one can get excited about improvement because even the smallest of improvements is inspirational. I understand that sexual violence will most likely always be around and "I" cannot change that but if I can contribute to significant improvement then that is something to stay inspired and passionate about.

In my own empirical research of sexual predators, I have found that several of them have been sociopaths. They have little-to-no moral conscious and they lack empathy and respect for rules, authority, and boundaries. This has a biological context because many sociopaths have been known to have smaller amygdalae than most people which limits their ability to empathize. <u>Not all sexual predators are sociopaths but the ones who are not tend to be influenced by a sociopathic mindset and attitude.</u> During lectures and discussion seminars I have given, I have used Polsky's Diamond to discuss this idea. Polsky's Diamond is a tool that can be used within groups to assess group dynamics.

> *"In his work, Pol sky described a hierarchy of power that he portrayed as a stratified diamond. The diamond suggests that the youth group hierarchy is not unlike that of most groups and organizations and can best be understood as a structure with little room at the top and the bottom and plenty of room in the middle. A few leaders and lieutenants (enforcers) fill the space at the top of the diamond, a few scapegoats and status seekers ("bush boys") are at the bottom, and most of the group members are in the middle. The leaders were usually the more intelligent youth in the group. The lieutenants were the physically strong individuals who carried out the leaders' orders. The middle group members were*

fundamentally followers. The status seekers were youth

looking for acceptance and upward mobility

(recognition); the scapegoats were the weak and

devalued persons," (Mullen, 1999).

Additionally, in Jon Ronson's book *THE PSYCHOPATH TEST*, he discusses the idea that many leaders of businesses and companies are actually psychopaths; encompassing sociopathic behavior. Regarding Polsky's Diamond you should notice the power and influence that the leaders have over the rest of the group. If the leaders are promoting a rape culture then guess what can happen? A rape culture is given life to. I bring this up to say that even though a status seeker or any non-leader who may not actually be a sociopath, in a way they are still influenced by a sociopathic mindset and attitude. It does not take accountability away from the non-leader for engaging in sexually violent acts but it does shed a non-traditional (and ignored) light on the roots of many types of violence.

So what are some of the solutions to killing sexual violence? Great question. We will cover that throughout the entire book, but let's start with social responsibility and your own sociopathy. Yes, YOU too have a certain level of sociopathy in you. We all do. Every human being, no matter how much you have convinced yourself of your own self-humility, empathy, and kindness, you too have the ability to exercise sociopathy; and it is very much needed in certain situations. It is the nature of war; *and fighting sexual violence is a war*. If you have two people in a fight and one person is willing to go to the extreme and the other person is not willing to meet or exceed the same extreme levels, this person is at a disadvantage. Though I do have empathy for sexual predators because they are in need of help as well due to some of them being victims of violent crimes, there are some people who are flat out evil and no longer have a desire to be helped; and you cannot reason with that type of sociopath. Good luck trying. One of the solutions in killing sexual violence is individuals within the culture and/or community (social responsibility) to utilize moral intentions with sociopathic capabilities. I consider sexual violence to be evil and if you look at a biblical character such as the arch angel Michael or a comic book super hero and shero, they have every intension to *make the world a better place* (moral intensions) but they are very capable of killing any evil in the way (sociopathic capabilities). They are courageous, fearless, and part sociopathic. I want to emphasize this sociopathic aspect because to live a life in the world without practicing situational apathy is ridiculous. **I am not promoting the idea for you to physically kill someone**. I am promoting the idea that you may have to display apathy and kill a potentially dangerous thought someone has, or firmly redirect a behavior of someone before it becomes their way of being or lifestyle. For example, my father was robustly against me hitting my sisters. I remember one of the first times I hit my little sisters he bent down to my eye level and said to me, "If I ever hear or see you hit your sisters again, I'm going to kick your fucking ass." I later found out that he was serious (lol) and hitting my sisters faded away quickly. He didn't care about my feelings or any of that. He displayed apathy and sociopathy and I began to believe in my mind that making a lifestyle out of hitting a female was *bad*. That may not be the universal truth but my father created the belief in my mind that being violent towards people, especially towards women, was something that was immoral. My father's efforts were to kill maladaptive belief systems in my mind. You may not be a fighter, yeller, screamer, etc. but there are many other ways to be authentically fearless. You can create poetry, music, literature, artwork, etc., that attack sexual violence. You can create exciting games for games systems that are just as exhilarating but not as distasteful as the taboo ones out there. Everyone does not have to fight as ground troops. We need some people in the air, in the water, we need spies on the inside, and of course we need our own snipers. If and when this occurs it will create global solidarity and social responsibility that will influence a *penetration* of evil cultures of concealment and help kill sexual violence.

Manhood

I remember a time in my childhood where I got the courage to question my father about my responsibilities in the house and why I had to do certain things. "Dad, why do I have to do this but the girls (my sisters) don't have to do it? How cum' I have to do all this stuff?" He said, "Because by the time you leave my house, I'm going to make sure that you're a man." I was thinking *Dude I'm 10 years old. I don't care about that stuff yet (lol)*. Fast forward to today, I do care about manhood and I am strongly unsatisfied with the state of masculinity. We have all of these messages around us about what men are and what they shouldn't be and rarely do they get challenged in a soulful way; especially when it comes to incorporating the female aspect of masculinity. Licensed clinical psychologist Dr. Ian Edwards promotes the idea that healthy masculinity includes some feminine qualities. Within the following subtitles of this chapter I am going to walk you through more effective strategies that my company PerspectVe LLC has been using to kill sexual violence via **redefining manhood**. Some of those ways are but not limited to

1) exploring the mindset and attitude of being a young person,

2) exploring – developmentally, the emotions and desires of males and how this is acted out within masculinity,

3) redefining manhood with an individualistic approach, and

4) creating and gaining an understanding of how "being in-love" enhances ones manhood while rejecting certain violent attitudes.

<u>BEING YOUNG</u>

I was on a television talk show with Dr. Edwards and we discussed masculinity with the incredible host Lynne Hayes-Freeland. Ian talked about taking a look at archetypes of not just men but people in-general. He stated that there are *layers* within every human being and in looking at the archetype of different types of people, it will unveil a great deal of information and can potentially provide us with the ability to renovate what lays within the individual; in this case sexual predators. With that said, let's cut into these layers and go deep into the area of *youth…*

When I think about the state of being young, some of the connotations that come to my mind are *immaturity, partying, craziness, drugs, sex, excessive fun,* etc. I also think about the word <u>invincible</u>. Many of the younger people I come across admit that there are times when they feel immune to life's hardships and humbling moments. If I am being transparent with myself, I felt like this all throughout my childhood up to the age of 21. During my previous job as an In-Home Specialist I was working with a kid in the Homewood section of Pittsburgh, Pa and he had been running away from home every week for three months. During this time there were a string of violent murders in the community and he did not seem to care about the danger involved in him running away and staying out all night. When I had a conversation with him he confirmed my assessment of the situation regarding his feeling of invincibility. He said, "When I leave my house at night and make it home in the morning and nothing happens to me, **I feel like I beat the game**." He was thrill seeking. This kid was living in a real life video game. When we all told him about the dangers of what he was doing or when he heard news stories about the murders that were occurring, he did not believe that they applied to him because he felt *invincible*. It is important to highlight this idea because <u>the feeling of invincibility along with other aspects of</u>

29

being young can create a culture that may produce attitudes that lead to [sexual] violence (think Polsky's Diamond). I write all of this to say that there is a connection between the desire to thrill-seek, psychosocial messages (particularly peer influence), [sexualized] images (television, magazines, etc.), early life experiences, and violence. Humans can be very impressionable in their youth. Therefore, in order to kill sexual violence, another method to slaughter it [early on] is to improve psychosocial development at an earlier age by

1) offering healthier messages and 2) encouraging true self-discovery among the youth, which I think is an *integral piece*. Improving the psychosocial condition and offering healthier messages are traditional ideas but the encouragement of self-discovery has been *ignored* for a long time. I believe self-discovery is a powerful part of the solution because ideologically our true sense of self may be one that has no space or tolerance for sexual violence. One could argue that on the continuum of life, ones true self could be evil – *and I would agree with that*. However (think about Polsky's Diamond again), if everyone in the group is engaging in self-discovery

and trying to be the best self possible, I postulate that the group dynamics change, possibly to the point where there is no group anymore, or the group is segmented into smaller groups. **If people are being true to themselves they can become leaders for themselves** because they are not as <u>impressionable</u> and victims of this top-down-effect (Polsky's Diamond). Even in the instance where the group still exists, if the leader at the top is someone with a positive influence, the group dynamics will look different and *the mindset of the group will not be one of malice, evil, and unnecessary violence.* In the movie THE EQUALIZER, Denzel Washington plays a sociopathic hero. He goes around killing noir men who are engaged in the pimping of women. My favorite line in that movie is when he says, "You gotta be who you [truly] are, right?" He's a sociopathic leader (top) who is endeared by the people around him (the group). He discovered *and accepted* his true self (which is partly sociopathic) and he is killing sexual predators. Imagine that…

<u>WHO TOLD YOU THAT?</u>

Unfortunately, many people enlist themselves to be representatives for the unhealthy psychosocial messages that pervade the human psyche (particularly the *masculine* psyche). I have no idea what the phrase <u>real man</u> means but when I have asked audiences to define it, some of the responses include paying the bills, being physically strong, winning fights, having multiple women, having sexual prowess, etc. The follow up question I ask is *who told you that!?!* I remember I was at a bar-b-q for one of my college buddies birthdays and his mother began getting very intoxicated and she told me that her husband has other women who he sleeps with and she said that she is not bothered by it at all. "Men are not supposed to be faithful to one woman," she stated. Continuing, "As long as he takes care of me I don't care what he does with other women." She represents this message and this is how psychosocial messages are perpetually birthed into the minds of people generation after generation. Whether her statement is her truth or not, my point is that *I do not have to accept that statement to be true for me*. The fact that I have engaged in soulful <u>self-discovery</u> and become a <u>leader for myself</u>, *her belief system cannot penetrate my belief system*.

On another occasion, a male that I endeared and had almost as much respect for as my own father told me after my wedding that it was ok to sleep with different women because *it's just what men do*. Even though I am a strong willed person and not impressionable by most people, I was affected by his statement because in this relationship I may have been the lieutenant; cautiously but potentially willing to follow his lead in some situations. For two weeks I felt confused about my decision to be faithful to my wife because a person who I thought of as supremely wise and empathetic of the serious marital union was encouraging me to cheat. I came to the conclusion that I do not have to be like most men. I can choose to be a different [arche]type of man. I can challenge these messages that people told me. *I can be a different representative.* I do not have to think like *the group* and believe what other people tell me.

BEING IN-LUST vs. BEING IN-LOVE

We have been lead to believe that the world needs more love. That is bullshit. Love is ubiquitous. It is around even if and when you think it is not. What the world needs is for more people to fall in-love. For example, there are colleges around the nation that are experiencing a decline in student enrollment. The college officials do not say "Let's build another college." They strategize ways to get more people in college. There is plenty of love in the universe but there is not a lot of people who are in-love. If there were more people in-love there may not be as much suffering in the world because the spirit of being in-love kills the desire to intentionally hurt those people and things in which one is in-love with. It does not mean that you cannot and will not hurt someone but what it can do is kill your conscious thought to do it *intentionally*. That is why love itself is sort of shitty. You can love someone and still intentionally hurt them and someone can love you and still intentionally hurt you. I loved some of my girlfriends of the past but I would still have sex with other girls (which hurt my girlfriend's feelings) simply because I was horny. It was a shitty thing to do and I take responsibility for my actions but at the time I was 1) influenced by the group (I surely was not a leader), 2) had not discovered my true self and 3) I was not in-love. When I accepted my true self for who I was and simultaneously fell in-love with my wife **and humanity**, there was no more room in my mind, body, spirit, and soul to accept and act out unhealthy messages and intentionally hurt people. Not only is this an elixir for sexual violence it is an elixir for violence".""

<u>SLUTS & BITCHES</u>

One of my favorite things about the Bloom's Sanctuary Model ® is the paradigm shift it causes when it promotes the idea that when looking at someone's behavior we should not ask *what is wrong with them?*, instead we should ask ourselves *what has happened to them?*. I have been guilty of calling women out of their name (including women in my own family). Though I have written extensively thus far about the impact of what culture and society does to us, *we must not blame the culture for things that **we decided** to take from it.* As you can tell I am a major proponent against sexual violence and though I do not believe that men are the only sexual predators, I think that women deserve increased empathy because statistically they are the ones more severely impacted by sexual violence than men.

I used to work with a young 16 year old female who we will call Vanessa. She was a physically beautiful young lady and a bit mature for her age. She had a negative reputation in the community that she lived in and she was known as the neighborhood slut. Vanessa was engaging in sexual activities with men in their mid-forties (over 20 years even my age at the time), skipping school, and riding with the neighborhood stick-up kids. Her mother was a young single mom herself in her early thirties and she had no idea what to do with her daughter anymore. Vanessa was being taunted by other girls in her school and many of the boys were targeting her for sex. What the people who were calling her names did not know was that four months previously, within a two-week span, Vanessa had three major traumatic experiences. She was raped, attacked on her way home from school, and a close family member passed away not too long after these incidents. These three things all happened within a matter of two weeks. The community didn't know this. The people bullying her at school didn't know this. All they knew was the behavioral result of her pain; inappropriate relationships with older men and community violence.

"Some victims of violent crimes become promiscuous and develop the idea that they enjoy sex because it's a defense mechanism in dealing with their own pain and suffering. It is easier to say 'I liked it' than to deal with the idea that maybe 'I didn't like it'," (Laurie Kessler, 2015).

Vanessa became clinically depressed and apathetic about life. During one particular therapy session she told me that she wanted to kill herself but she could not bring herself to actually doing it. And because she stopped caring about living, she also stopped caring about herself. When opportunities arose to engage in unhealthy activities (and there were plenty) she had no apprehensions because she did not want to be alive. Her attitude was *Why not sleep with these men? Why not go rob people? What else is there to do? What do I have to live for?* I personally believe that part of her was hoping that someone would do to her what she could not do to herself; *kill her.* Many people in her community were wondering what was wrong with her but no one ever thought to reflect on what may have happened to her. She did not wake up one day and randomly decide to become sexually promiscuous or a young criminal. She was behaving in a maladaptive way because she was a little girl who was raped, beaten within inches of her life, and saw a family member who she loved get murdered… *all within two weeks.* No one seemed to be interested in checking in with her to ask her "Hey Vanessa, what's been going on? What's happened to you?" They did not think about the idea that hurt people hurt people. She was hurt and she began hurting other people in the world, including herself. If you do not ever contribute large amounts of your energy to help kill sexual violence, one of the least of things that you can do that would have a huge effect towards killing sexual violence is to be understanding of people that have had some horrific things happen to them and to display empathy for them as wounded people even when they act out excessively.

Can You Tell I'm A Predator/Perpetrator?

My career has been built on being transparent. However, sometimes one must use selective transparency for the sake of the greater good and in this chapter I will exercise just that, *selective transparency*. I will not speak in depth about how to identify a sexual predator/perpetrator but I do encourage you to recognize themes in the things you read about them, similarities in how their victims have described them, etc. My goal is not to cloak the information. I am simply being strategic in how I choose to engage in the art of war. In previous pages, I have provided some key elements in the fight to kill sexual violence but not every weapon needs to be showed and discussed in view of those people who may potentially use it to inflict further harm which would go against the greater goal. After all, it is unwise to show the people on the other team your strategy; if you plan to win.

If you can gain an increased understanding in how to assess sexual predators/perpetrators, you can gain a significantly increased ability in keeping yourself and those around you safe. Sexual predators/perpetrators come in all sizes, shapes, and forms, and are in all walks of life. This can also include your family and friends. Do not underestimate the evil of the people within your own familial and social network. Many rape victims report being sexually assaulted and/or raped by the people they know, not a stranger. Here is something that needs to be stated, that many men – who are trying to be respectfully helpful to victims, supportive, and tactfully honest, get in trouble for addressing; *in addition to gaining awareness about sexual predators, it is paramount for people (both male and female) to become aware how not to become the victims of sexual predators.* You will not be the cool guy in the room if you tell a rape and sexual assault victim that it was their fault for getting assaulted. It may be true that some people (women in particular) fantasize about being subdued via rough sex but I highly doubt that there are people begging for someone to rape them. In order to put sexual violence six feet under the ground, people need to not become targets. I am not insinuating that women have to *dress different* but I am seriously requesting that all people be mindful of how they may or may not contribute to a dangerous situation. I reviewed a study regarding sexual violence that was done at a university in Pittsburgh, Pa and I could not believe one particular segment of the data. One of the surveys asked female students which activities they prefer engaging in on Friday and Saturday evenings. Over 80% of them stated clubbing, dancing, and drinking. Then, it asked them at which point throughout their week and where did they feel the most unsafe and likely to be sexually assaulted. Nearly the same percentage of students said <u>on Friday and Saturday nights when they are out</u> *socializing*. Please excuse my language when I write *WTF*. This is a prime example of what I mean in describing the nature of feeling **young and invincible**. These students, in a way, are consciously contributing to potential risk, whether the risk is actual or only in their own psyche. I do not want to tell anyone not to party and have a fun time but if your partying and fun come with an increased feeling of being the victim of violence, maybe you should reevaluate your definition of fun and the places and people you choose to have fun with. I encourage everyone to have fun; but be smart.

Though I am not going to show my full hand, I do encourage you to find creative ways to figure out patterns and phenomenological consistencies among sexual

predators/perpetrators, not because they are going to hurt you

but so that you can put your focus in not contributing to being

hurt by them.

SIGHT AND SEX – *Talking to the sexual predator.*

Can I tell you something? I used to be one of the world's best womanizers. I LOVED partying with pretty girls my age and older women. Breast, thighs, pretty face and all of that; I loved them being in my presence. And I still appreciate a beautiful female specimen. If I see a pretty women, do I look at her briefly and allow my eyes to briefly assess her? You're damn right I do! Why wouldn't I acknowledge a great piece of human artistry that the Higher Power created? Sexual stimulation, horniness, physical attraction, or whatever you want to call it is part of the human experience. To deny or block oneself from experiencing it is actually unhealthy. I am a faithful one-woman man who is happily married and a robust proponent of monogamous relationships. To what may be your surprise, I do not believe that monogamous relationships are normal but I do believe that they are healthier. We are attracted to different people for different reasons, even if it is outside of our intimate relationship with the person who we are in-love with but just because something is natural does not mean that it is ok to act upon or act out. It is believed that philosopher Epictetus once said that *freedom is not fulfillment of your desires, it is removal of them.* I am a very strong believer of that idea but I also believe that there is great freedom in not trying to eliminate the desire (which may be unhuman) but to overcome the additional desire of acting out other desires. I talk a lot about killing the desire to sexually violate people and from a marketing PerspectVe it is great. It has a shock value to it and it gets people's attention. Realistically, as I have previously stated, some things will not go away; and unhealthy desires may be one of them. Sex is one of the most powerful forces within the universe, and though I have not ever experienced the desire to sexually violate someone else for any reason, other people have – and that desire may not ever be able to be killed.

What can be killed are any successive desires to act out those unhealthy root desires. When I see a beautiful woman my mind may become *imaginative*. I may undress her in mind, I may fantasize about what her intimacy might be like, etc. I acknowledge the sexual thoughts that temporarily pervade my mind and I let them go. Since I have invested and created a fulfilling lifestyle that meets my needs, combined with the belief in no-belief in sexual violence, I have killed any chance of me acting on any lustful desires outside of my relationship with my wife no matter how natural they are. *I have won the battle of mind vs. behavior.* **What occurs in my mind does not have to occur in my behavioral life.** To Epictetus's point, there is a great freedom and power in discipline – especially sexual discipline. At the age of 24 I serendipitously stumbled upon sexual discipline and I did not ever think it was something that was possible for me. When I became increasingly sexually disciplined, I achieved ongoing highs and phenomenal experiences in my life that are nearly unexplainable. There is a common belief that sexual violence is all about power and though I do not believe that, my message to a sexual predator is that if you think sexually violating someone is powerful, overcoming that desire can take you to a new level of spiritual and holistic power that you may not have ever known existed. At a minimum you will discontinue malicious acts of sexual violence on people, but there are potentially more gifts for you for overcoming that desire that will not just create a better world for others but a better internal world for YOU. To any sexual predator that may be reading this book, I do not like what you do and I am very serious about killing sexual violence in whatever way necessary. Though I am disgusted with some of your actions in life, I empathize with your soul because I myself am not perfect either.

I was taking notes during a discussion I had with Dr. Edwards and he educated me about his philosophy of what he believes is one way to move from human to human violence to empathy for the fellow human. He says that ignorance leads to objectivizing someone which then leads to violence. He then states that compassion leads to making a person a subject which then leads to empathy. How awesome is that!?! Even though I love this idea, my only objection to it is that I believe it only applies to people who have a normal and/or increased ability to empathize; which eliminates many sociopaths. I do believe that the sociopath can learn empathy and compassion in the same way that they learned evil and malice, but it takes more work. It also takes an environment (i.e. an appropriate household) that will challenge sociopathic tendencies. For example, licensed professional counselor, Dr. Matthew Walsh states, "People may have the genetic make up to become a sociopath but the environmental factors can prevent the activation of those characteristics," (Walsh, 2016). But since many sociopaths are extremely impulsive and may not have had an appropriate upbringing, it is easier for them to accept a life of darkness and grim rather than to overcome those instincts towards living a fulfilling life of self-love and happiness. **In order to kill sexual violence there must be a psychological suicide of the sexual predatory psyche in order for a rebirth of an improved psyche**.

References

(1985-2016). Retrieved from The Sanctuary Model:
    http://www.sanctuaryweb.com/TheSanctuaryModel.aspx

Kirby, P. (2012). Refusing to be a Man?: Men's Responsibility for War Rape
    and the Problem of Social Structures in Feminist and Gender Theory.
    Brighton, United Kingdom. Retrieved from
    http://r.search.yahoo.com/_ylt=A0LEVickJ9BXAicAQJsnnIlQ;_ylu=
    X3oDMTByOHZyb21tBGNvbG8DYmYxBHBvcwMxBHZ0aWQD
    BHNlYwNzcg--
    /RV=2/RE=1473288101/RO=10/RU=https%3a%2f%2fthedisorderoft
    hings.files.wordpress.com%2f2014%2f06%2fkirby-paul-2013-
    refusing-to-be-a-man.pdf/

Laurie Kessler, Phd. (2015). Sexual Violence Discussion. (S. Coleman,
    Interviewer)

McClellan, S. (2008). *WHAT HAPPENED - Inside the Bush White House and
    Washington's Culture of Deception.* New York: Public Affairs.

Mullen, J. (1999). Retrieved from ProQuest:
    http://search.proquest.com/docview/214196371?pq-origsite=gscholar

Walsh, D. M. (2016, October 2016). Sociopaths & Sexual Violence. (S. Coleman,
    Interviewer)

WHO. (2016). *Violence against women - Intimate partner and sexual violence
    against women.* Retrieved from
    http://www.who.int/mediacentre/factsheets/fs239/en/

REDEFINING MANHOOD
Addressing sexual violence and rape
culture in a way *no one else will.*

"It helped me to rethink how I think about women before I act."

"Very thought-provoking and [it] encouraged good dialogue between myself and my brothers."

"All the brothers seemed to take away a lot from this [discussion]."

"I thought it was very interesting and thought provoking and gives you a different perspective of how to see women."

These are some of the things that fraternity members and males in general have been saying after the seminar discussions I have been doing at high schools and university campuses. In 2003 I turned 18 years of age and became a legal adult, but it was not until the age of 23 that I believe I began to enter into true manhood. As I have continued to reflect on the topic itself, I must say – I'm thoroughly disgusted with the state of masculinity and what continues to be projected and encouraged from some. High school after high school, college after college, and place after place I continue to hear and read how males and females define manhood and it is alarming. The onus is not completely on them because many of these messages have been written onto our Tabula Rasa thanks to psychosocial

51

development. Since self-discovery is not promoted within some cultures, these maladaptive messages become the embedded foundations that create our belief systems about manhood.

I am also sickened by the strategies that are being used to "attack and eliminate" unhealthy behaviors in both males **and females** – because this is not solely a male issue. I attended a conference lead by a well-respected colleague who travels internationally fighting against sex slavery. It was a very informative and poignant presentation. She talked about how billions of dollars are being spent to educate people on the topic and rescue missions are being completed to save women. Great stuff. Inspirational! I enjoyed it. But I noticed that there was no talk about addressing the male desire to assault, rape, and violate women. So I raised my hand and asked "Is there any action being taken to address the male desire to engage in these violent types of sexual behaviors?" She paused and searched for an answer, looking a bit flustered, then stuttered a little bit and said "Well no…there's no task force or money being spent to address that." So you are telling me that billions of dollars are being spent to educate people, save women, and do other admirable things but nothing is being done to address **the core issue**!?! If that is the case then we have a major problem. It's as if a boxer is going out to fight just for the sake of fighting. He has no real strategy, doesn't really know much about his opponent, has not trained well, but expects to win – and has been doing this his entire career.

My discontentment and anger came to an all-time high in mid-2015 when I was serendipitously talking to a mentor of mine, who is a psychologist that shared some of the same views as me. He had attended a couple previous unrelated seminars I had done and he thought I was the right person to address these issues. He summoned me to put together a seminar that is discussion-based and that addresses manhood, sexual violence, and rape culture in a non-traditional way while being non-judgmental towards the audience. The results? *Incredible!* Not only have these discussions been educational, exciting, and fun; **young and older men are actually saying that they want to become more aware of their unhealthy thoughts towards women so that they can challenge these thoughts**. It has gotten to the point where staff members at the events and audience members follow up before we get a chance to follow up with them. *What's the secret you ask?* Well, without giving away the full recipe, some of the salient ingredients have been 1 cup of non-traditional advertisement, 2 cups of tactful courage, and a great product!

We hope to help your establishment with any needs you may have and WE HOPE you can help us continue to redefine manhood by addressing sexual violence and rape culture in a way no one else will.

For booking please use the information below:
PerspectVe LLC
(412)592-2291
www.PerspectVe.com
PerspectVeLLC@yahoo.com

Is it humane to RAPE someone?

People tell me "Shawn, you're a good guy."..."If only there were more people in the world like you." I was even approached one random afternoon while crossing the street after a college graduation by a person who confessed to being a physic. Even as a therapist, that was a very awkward encounter for me to have; a stranger approach me and know things about me as if they were a lifelong friend or family member. Before she parted she said "Shawn, you're a good man." Compliments are fine and most people enjoy them. I am not one of those people. I appreciate these kind words when they are given to me and I understand that the appreciation other people have for me when they offer their endearment. I'm thankful for it and I would not tell people not to do it because it is a gift they want to give you. Most of the time, I just feel like I don't need the compliments. Plus, as one of the deities teaches, *no man or woman is good*. I am a *decent* human being. I desire to be true to myself. My true self just happens to me someone who desires to display as much morality, love, faith in God as possible and give off healthy energy. But please believe *I am human*. There

55

are things about me that are not good and are not

descent. Unfortunately (and maybe fortunately) I have been in

situations in my life to where I have showed myself that I can

behave in what may be considered evil, horrid, and

heartless. This is a very small part of me but it is still a part of

me. I strongly postulate that you have displayed similar

qualities too. Believe it or not, it is more human than you

think. But here's my question, does the fact (or *theory*) that

evilness is part of being human make it ok to engage in evil

ways?

I use to involve myself with many aggressive people

and activities; some of those people and activities still present in

my life today. However, the people have matured and the

activities are in sublimated forms. For as much violence,

aggression, and rage that I inflicted on other people during

physical altercations and also had inflicted upon me, it is

difficult for me to wrap my head around the idea that it is ok to

do these things to a child, a handicap person, a mentally

challenged individual, a woman, etc. Not to insinuate that

harming a man is ok but what type of authentic or true human believes it is ok to harm someone simply because they can (especially a vulnerable being no matter the gender)? And my salient question, what type of human develops the desire to rape another person? A debater may say *Well Shawn, you said that evil is part of being human. Anybody is capable of this.* Yes, thanks to trauma that is true. I am well aware of the impact that trauma has on the human psyche and how hurt people hurt people (thus helping create evil). I am also aware of the power of sex and lust. I am aware of all of this but it does not negate the idea of what a respected peer of mine encourages in the idea of being able to use TRUE POWER to overcome evil, lustful, hurtful, and unhealthy desires. I read a lot of literature about sexual violence, rape, and other aggressive behaviors and they indicate that the aggressive act is about gaining power. I am not in total agreement with that idea. That is not true power. That is abdicating ones power, succumbing to and being enslaved by the desire. True power is being able to acknowledge the desire and overcome it. That is a powerful feeling! You may be thinking *Why didn't you overcome your own aggressive desires to fight?* My response is that they were not desires. My aggressive behaviors were a response to my external surroundings more than they were an inner desire to inflict harm upon another being. Even back in my more aggressive years, I would have always opted to avoid any situation regarding someone else's detriment because that is not the type of person I am.

In accordance with the title of this blog and the state of rape and sexual violence (R&SV) [towards women in particular], the problem with R&SV is that there is a male desire to rape and sexually violate women. I am continually appalled to see a lack of people understanding this. If you want to significantly reduce R&SV towards eradicating it, one of the goals needs to be attacking the desire to engage in these inappropriate behaviors towards others. In the world of sex slavery and prostitution, Linda Smith and Cindy Coloma write,

> *"Without a buyer, there wouldn't be a seller and there wouldn't be a victim. The demand for commercial sexual services fuels the problem of domestic minor sex trafficking....And so – to understand clearly – we have to go back to the beginning. To the 'why' of*

prostitution. It's simple supply and demand. There is a buyer who wants a product," (Coloma & Smith, 2013).

Trauma, evil, and a multitude of unfortunate factors create the harsh reality that rape and sexual violence will occur and they also give us a glimpse into how some individuals are pervaded by these unhealthy desires. But it does not stave off the reality that people need help to overcome their evil ways.

We hope to help your establishment with any needs you may have in addressing this unhealthy type of mentality.

For booking please use the information below:
PerspectVe LLC
(412)592-2291
www.PerspectVe.com
PerspectVeLLC@yahoo.com

References
Coloma, L. S. (2013). *RENTING LACY - A Story of America's Prostituted Children.* Vancouver: Shared Hope International .

I thank you for reading! You can reach me at www.PerspectVe.com. Remember to spell the word PerspectVe without the "i" because to broaden your own horizons, sometimes you have to take yourself out of your own PerspectVe. Take care and I pray you a happy, healthy, and meaningful life of success, and fulfillment through God.

Other Books by the Author

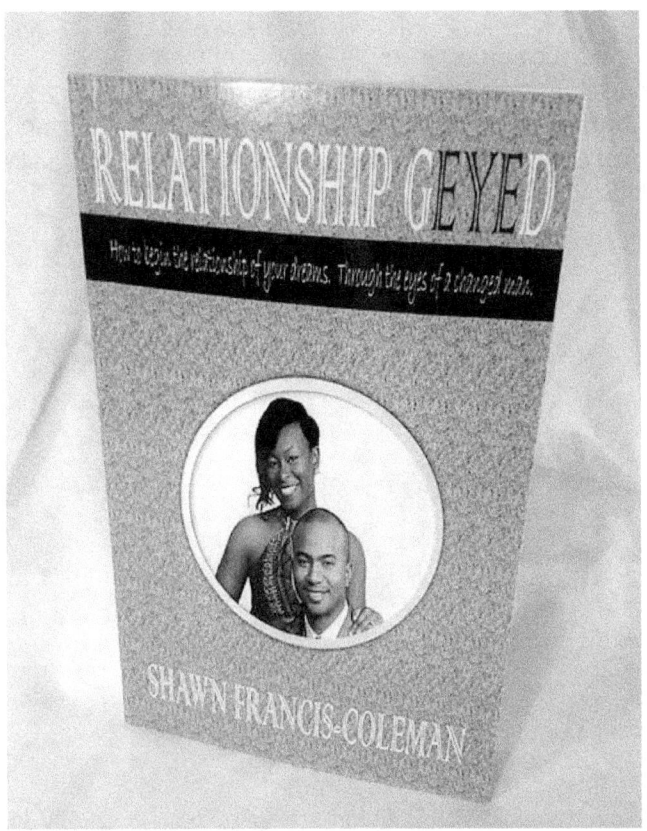

RELAITONSHIP GEYED - This book tells the true story about a period in one man's life when he met a woman whose behavior and lifestyle inspired him to leave his life of inappropriate relationships with other women, partying, violence, and self-destruction. Continuing to reap the benefits of being happy and in-love years later, while hearing so many other people cry and anger about their relationship situation, the author was propelled to share 13 unique elements that influenced him to become a faithful one-woman-man in a fairy-tale-like relationship.

With each chapter readers will not only find themselves emotionally invested and entertained by the author's transparent style of writing, they will gain an increased ability to improve multiple areas of their relationship life.

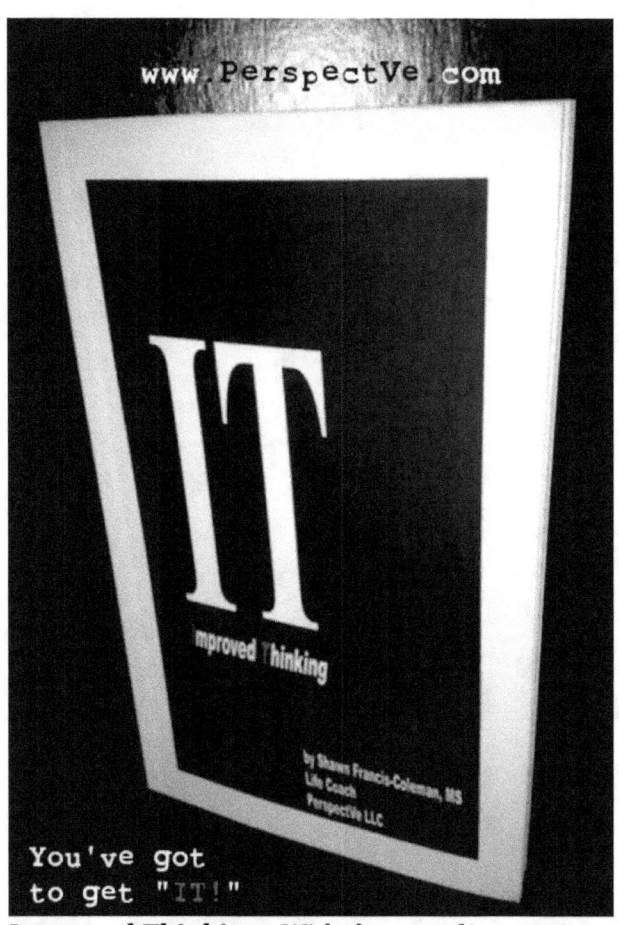

Improved Thinking - With the use of innovative quotes/philosophies, and therapeutic boxing quotes/philosophies, IT provides a new and improved way of thinking that will expand your PerspectVe™ concerning different areas of life. While paying homage to famous quotes from Les Brown, Gandhi, Helen Keller, Mark Twain, Bruce Lee and many more, this book builds on philosophies of the past and present and positions to be the next generation of quotes and philosophies in its own right.

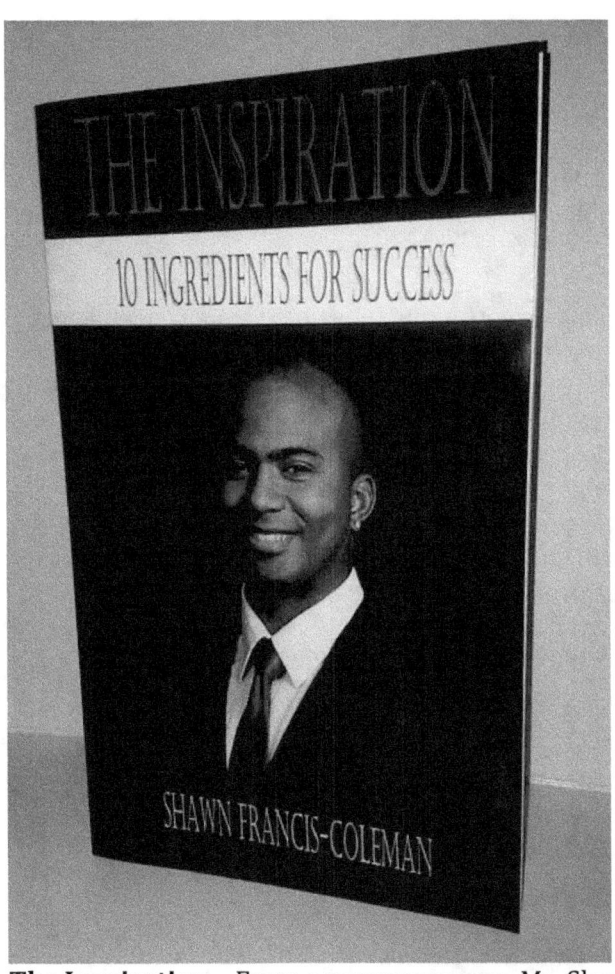

The Inspiration – From a very young age, Mr. Shawn Coleman has had the opportunity to meet high profile individuals locally and globally. He met the greatest basketball player to have ever lived, rubbed shoulders with world renowned musicians, and was surrounded with a village of people that included family, friends, and other incredible individuals from different walks of life. Though Shawn struggled with some serious personal issues as a young man, he never passed up the chance to interview the successful people he was around and he always inquired about their journey to success. As he got older and began to research other successful people, he noticed 10 ingredients that were being used by nearly every successful person he spoke to.

After seven years of meeting with popular people and studying the practices and behaviors of other successful people, Mr. Coleman wrote this book to help other people on the road to success regardless of the time period. He illustrates each ingredient of success by using real life inspirational stories that give each chapter their own individual character that are brought to life. Readers will find this short text to be just as powerful as other famous self-help books but they will discover different intimate treasures that are applicable to their own individual goals and desires and not generalized to every reader. More success awaits you...get to reading!

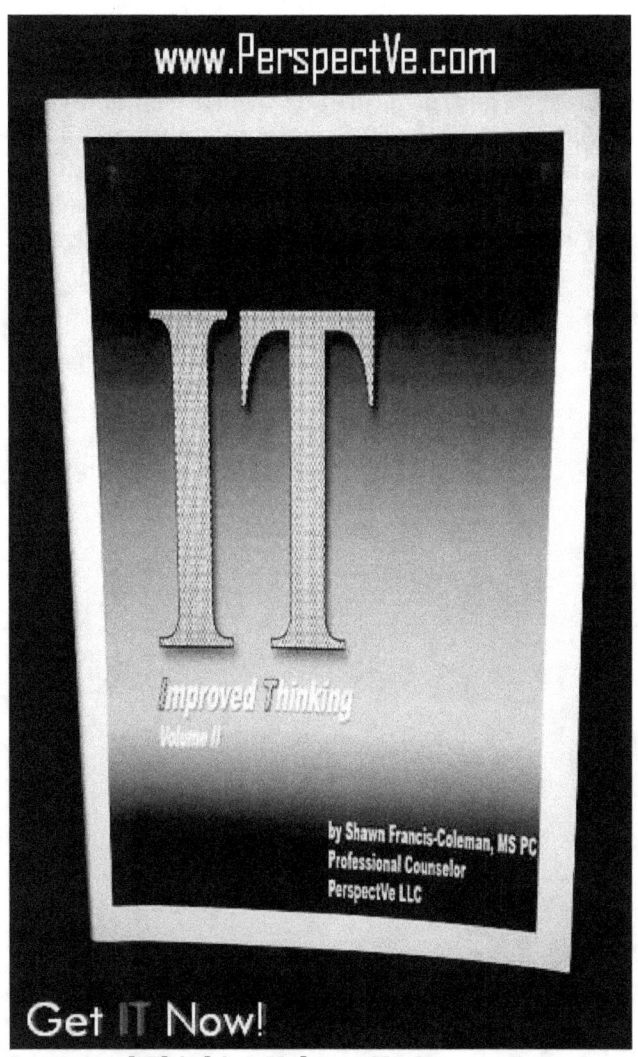

Improved Thinking Volume II - In a continuation of the first edition of this book, I have provided you with 300 more inspirational quotes, philosophies, and ideas that I pray help you within various aspects of your life and encourage you to live powerful! Like the first volume, I give you 300 new pieces of my mind in the form of literary artwork. As you read through each page, let your mind travel to a relatable experience (past, present, and/or future) that you are familiar with.   As your mind, body, spirit, soul, emotions, and behaviors align, take notice of how the Improved Thinking within this book will improve your quality of life and well-being. Have a great journey in the pages to come and I hope that you get IT!...Improved Thinking that is...

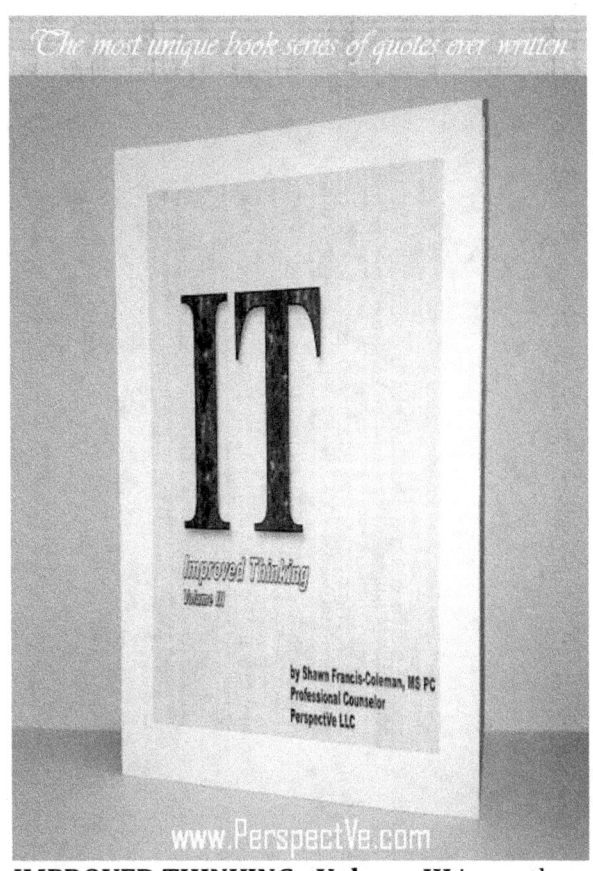

IMPROVED THINKING - Volume III is another exhilarating experience that will expand your worldview of your external and internal universe. It will provide you with non-traditional concepts that will increase your ability to live within a healthier and happier you!